Hair growth

21 HERB'S FOR HAIR GROWTH

Olivia peters

Table of contents

Here are 21 herbs that can make your hair grow

Chapter 1

Rosemary

A common herb that is known to encourage hair development is rosemary oil. Usually, it is combined with other carrier oils like coconut or olive oil as an essential oil.

Rosemary oil has several advantages, one of which is that it delays hair aging. Additionally, it promotes healthy hair development by treating diseases like dandruff and soothing a dry, flaky scalp.

.

Chapter 2

Peppermint

Another conventional herbal therapy for treating hair loss and promoting hair growth in people is peppermint oil. It functions by stimulating hair growth by enhancing hair follicle proliferation.

Additionally, it promotes the scalp's blood flow and aids in holding the hair roots to the scalp. Because of its antifungal and anti-inflammatory qualities, peppermint is a popular remedy for itching and inflammation.

As a growth promoter, peppermint oil is normally diluted and applied to the scalp and hair. The increased blood flow increases the nutrition received by hair follicles, encouraging hair growth.

Chapter 3

Aloe vera

Any hair or skincare routine should include aloe vera gel. It supports a pH that is balanced and healthy, which encourages healthy hair development.

In addition to halting hair loss and encouraging nutrition, the gel functions as a natural conditioner. For optimum results, directly apply the aloe vera gel to your scalp and hair. Then, let it work its magic.

Chapter 4

Nettle

A well-known plant called nettle can assist with hair loss issues. It functions by stimulating the scalp, enhancing blood flow, and preventing further deterioration and breakdown.

Nettle can be taken orally as tablets or as a rinse made from the powdered leaves and olive oil. This may lessen hair loss and encourage healthy hair growth.

.

Chapter 5

Ginkgo Biloba

It's about time you learned about this amazing plant if you haven't already. Not only is this plant good for the skin, but it also promotes hair development.

It increases blood flow and circulation throughout the body, which promotes thick, healthy hair growth.

It is also thought to support clearer skin. Ginkgo Biloba pills are an excellent choice for anyone looking to restore the health of their hair because several studies have shown that they successfully treat hair follicle deficits.

Chapter 6

Moringa

The thiocyanate-rich plant moringa strengthens hair follicles and reduces hair loss. It functions as a natural conditioner and encourages the development of new hair.

Use moringa powder to make a tea to rinse your hair, or use the oil form to apply straight to your hair. The health of your hair may be improved naturally and successfully with the help of this plant.

Chapter 7

Lavender

With its velvet-pink blooms, lavender not only looks beautiful, but it also has several advantages for the health of your hair.

Lavender works wonders to clear up bacterial or fungal problems and soothe the scalp. You may combine lavender essential oils with your preferred carrier oil, such as coconut or olive oil.

Lavender tea can enhance general health and promote healthy hair in addition to topical application. A multipurpose plant like lavender can improve your hair-care regimen.

Chapter 8

Rose petals

By creating a rinse with hot water, rose petals may be utilized to stimulate hair development and refresh hair.

They can also offer a healthy sheen and condition the hair. Rose petals can be used to heal irritated scalp because of their antibacterial qualities.

Chapter 9

Burdock

This plant is a potent weapon against hair loss and soothes an itchy, burning scalp thanks to its richness of fatty acids and phytosterol components. It works well to cure ailments like psoriasis and promote hair growth.

Chapter 10

Saw palmetto

Because saw palmetto and stinging nettle are related, combining the two can be quite successful in halting hair loss and encouraging hair growth.

Combining these herbs can promote new hair development and decrease the overproduction of DHT, a hormone associated with hair loss. This may lead to hair that is thicker and healthier.

Chapter 11

Ginseng

A popular Chinese plant called ginseng is a natural treatment for a number of health problems, including hair loss. Because it strengthens and nourishes the hair, it successfully combats balding and encourages hair growth. Numerous shampoos and hair tonics use ginseng as a main component.

Chapter 12

Coat buttons

Although this herb's name may be silly, its advantages for hair are not. When paired with other complimentary herbs, the Ayurvedic herb coat buttons, which is a high source of antioxidants, can help increase hair growth

Chapter 13

Brahmi

The herb known as brahmi, also known as bacopa monnieri, is well known for encouraging hair growth. It is frequently used in hair supplements and medications, and when mixed with other herbs for hair development, it works best.

Alkaloids, active proteins that promote hair development, are abundant in brahmi.

Chapter 14

Gooseberry (Amla)

This herb is a well-known Ayurvedic treatment for accelerating hair development and fortifying hair to stop breaking and hair loss.

Antioxidants found in abundance in it aid in the removal of free radicals that can harm hair follicles and cause hair loss. The herb's name is Bhringraj, and because of its many health advantages, it has long been utilized in traditional medicine.

Iron, magnesium, calcium, and vitamin E are among the vital minerals found in gooseberry that are naturally occurring and crucial for promoting healthy hair development.

These nutrients strengthen the hair strands, encourage proper blood circulation, and nourish the hair follicles.

The anti-inflammatory characteristics of bhringraj assist to calm the scalp, lessen irritation, and shield against head lice and dandruff.

Typically, the herb is administered topically in the form of a hair mask or oil. Regular usage can enhance the length, thickness, and general health of your hair. It is also thought to aid in preventing hair from prematurely graying.

Chapter 15

Jatamansi

The Ayurvedic herb jatamansi, sometimes referred to as spikenard, is well-known for its therapeutic benefits. It has rhizomes that have been shown to accelerate hair development and fortify hair, avoiding breaking and hair loss.

The herb's anti-inflammatory effects aid in calming the scalp and guard against fungal infections, dandruff, and other scalp irritations. Additionally enhancing blood flow to the scalp, jatamansi encourages hair growth.

Additionally, it is well recognized for helping hair regrow following chemotherapy treatments.

Chapter 16

Chinese hibiscus

Chinese hibiscus, often referred to as Hibiscus rosa sinensis, is a kind of hibiscus plant that promotes healthy hair development in addition to being tasty.

It has been shown that consuming Chinese hibiscus tea stimulates hair follicles, improving hair development and expanding hair follicle size.

As a result, it is a widely used component in a variety of hair care treatments, particularly those that promote thicker, longer hair.

Chapter 17

Green tea

Green tea is a renowned natural plant with many health advantages. It is stacked with panthenol, which fortifies hair, and antioxidants to help prevent hair loss.

Due to its advantageous qualities, it is a well-liked and successful remedy for hair damage and balding.

Chapter 18

Horsetail

Horsetail is a plant that can do wonders for your hair, despite its absurd name. Due to its high silica concentration, it is frequently featured in hair products since it strengthens hair, reduces hair loss and breakage, and enhances bone health.

You may buy hair products that contain horsetail as a key ingredient or take it as a supplement.

Horsetail is a diuretic plant, thus it's important to keep in mind that it might cause dehydration. Drink a lot of water when using horsetail to avoid this and safely enjoy its advantages.

Chapter 19

Bitter apple

Colocynth, commonly known as bitter apple, is a natural plant that has been used for generations as a medicine, particularly to encourage hair growth and stop hair loss.

The plant has qualities that energize hair follicles, which promote hair growth. Additionally, it has a lot of antioxidants, which lessen the likelihood of hair loss by preventing hair and scalp damage.

You may consume bitter apples in a variety of ways, such as as an oil, a tea, or a powder combined with other natural herbs.

Bitter apples can be rubbed into the scalp as a lubricant to increase blood flow and stimulate hair follicles.

The plant may also be made into a tea that can be consumed or used as a hair rinse. Alternatives include used as a conditioner or hair mask when combined with other herbs.

Chapter 20

Giant dodder

Ayurvedic medicine uses a plant called giant dodder to treat alopecia brought on by steroid hormones. This is because it has the potential to block the enzyme 5a reductase, which prevents testosterone from being converted into dihydrotestosterone (DHT), a hormone that promotes hair loss.

For the greatest effects, giant dodder is frequently used in conjunction with other herbs.

Chapter 21

Holy basil

Ocimum sanctum, sometimes referred to as holy basil, is a fragrant plant with several therapeutic benefits that can help alleviate irritation and hair loss.

It may work especially well for hair loss brought on by hormonal fluctuations or dandruff.

www.ingramcontent.com/pod-product-compliance
Lightning Source LLC
Chambersburg PA
CBHW060912260726

48661CB00008B/3599